Embracing the Storm

Navigating Depression, Anxiety and Anger During Menopause

By Gillianne Fuller

Copyright 2023 Gillianne Fuller for Menopause Matter

All rights reserved no part of this publication may be reproduced, distributed or transmitted in any form or by any means, including photocopying, recording or other electronic or mechanical method without the prior written permission of the publisher, except in the case of brief quotations embodied in critical reviews and certain other non-commercial uses permitted by copyright laws

ISBN 978-1-7782130-9-0

Published by: COJ Bookz
Cover by: S Bishop
Edited by: Desna Joy
Formatted By: Samiahmed321

www.menopausematter.org

Proceeds from the sale of the book goes to
Menopause Matter

Table Of Contents

INTRODUCTION 1
DEPRESSION 3
ANGER 31
DEALING WITH YOUR ANGER 37
ANXIETY 47
Conclusion 54
References 55

Gillianne Fuller for Menopause Matter

INTRODUCTION

Menopause is a natural process that marks the end of a woman's reproductive years. While some women experience a relatively smooth transition, others struggle with a range of physical and emotional symptoms that can affect their overall quality of life. Among these symptoms, depression, anger, and anxiety can be particularly challenging.

In this book, we will explore the unique challenges that women face during menopause, including the impact of hormonal changes on mental health. We will delve into the ways in which depression, anger, and anxiety can manifest during menopause, and offer practical strategies for managing these symptoms.

Our goal is to provide women with the tools and resources they need to navigate this important life transition with confidence and resilience. We believe that by understanding the physiological and emotional changes associated with menopause, women can make informed decisions about their health and well-being.

Whether you are experiencing depression, anger, or anxiety during menopause, or simply want to learn more about this important life transition, this book is for you. We invite you to join us on this journey and discover the power of knowledge, self-awareness, and self-care in managing menopausal symptoms and enhancing your overall health and happiness.

"Embracing the Storm: Navigating Depression, Anxiety, and Anger During Menopause"

Gillianne Fuller for Menopause Matter

DEPRESSION

Depression during menopause is a significant concern for many women, as hormonal changes and other factors can increase the risk of experiencing depressive symptoms.

The cause of depression during menopause is multifactorial and involves a combination of hormonal, physical, and psychosocial factors.

Some key factors contributing to depression in menopause include:

Hormonal changes: The primary cause of depression during menopause is the fluctuation and decline in hormone levels, particularly estrogen. Estrogen has been shown to play a role in mood regulation by influencing the production and function of neurotransmitters such as serotonin, norepinephrine, and dopamine. As estrogen levels decline during menopause, these neurotransmitters can be affected, potentially leading to depressive symptoms.

Menopausal symptoms: The physical symptoms of menopause, such as hot flashes, night sweats, and sleep disturbances, can significantly impact a woman's quality of life and contribute to the development of depression. Chronic sleep deprivation, for example, can exacerbate mood disturbances and increase the risk of depression.

Life stressors: Menopause often coincides with various life stressors, such as aging, changes in family dynamics, loss of fertility, and concerns about health and appearance. These stressors can increase the risk of depression during menopause, particularly for women who may already be prone to mood disorders.

Personal history: Women with a personal or family history of depression or other mental health disorders are at a higher risk of developing depression during menopause. Additionally, women who have experienced premenstrual dysphoric disorder (PMDD) or postpartum depression may also be more susceptible to depression during menopause.

Lifestyle factors: A sedentary lifestyle, poor diet, and lack of social support can also contribute to the development of depression during menopause.

It's important to recognize that the cause of depression in menopause is complex and may involve a combination of factors unique to each individual. Early identification and intervention are crucial in managing depression during menopause, and women experiencing depressive symptoms should seek help from a healthcare professional to develop an appropriate treatment plan.

HORMONAL CHANGES

Hormonal changes during menopause refer to the fluctuations and decline in the levels of female reproductive hormones, primarily estrogen and progesterone. These changes occur as a woman's ovaries gradually produce fewer hormones, leading to the cessation of menstruation and the end of her reproductive years. Hormonal changes during menopause can contribute to depression for several reasons:

Estrogen and mood regulation: Estrogen has been shown to play a role in mood regulation by influencing the production and function of neurotransmitters such as serotonin, norepinephrine, and dopamine. These neurotransmitters are crucial for maintaining stable mood and emotional well-being. As estrogen levels decline during menopause, the balance of these neurotransmitters can be disrupted, potentially leading to depressive symptoms.

Estrogen and stress response: Estrogen also helps modulate the body's stress response by regulating the production of cortisol, the primary stress hormone. When estrogen levels decrease during menopause, the stress response may become dysregulated, increasing a woman's vulnerability to stress and depression.

Interaction with other menopausal symptoms: The hormonal changes during menopause can also cause a range of physical symptoms, such as hot flashes, night sweats, and sleep disturbances. These symptoms can negatively impact a woman's quality of life, leading to increased stress, anxiety, and ultimately, depression.

It is essential to recognize that the relationship between hormonal changes and depression during menopause is complex and may involve various factors unique to each individual. Some women may be more sensitive to hormonal fluctuations, while others may be more resilient to these changes. Additionally, factors such as genetics, lifestyle, and overall health can influence the risk of depression during menopause.

If you suspect that hormonal changes during menopause are contributing to depressive symptoms, it's crucial to consult with a healthcare professional. They can help determine the underlying causes and develop an appropriate treatment plan.

SYMPTOMS

Depression during menopause can manifest in various symptoms, which may be similar to those experienced in depression at other times. Some common symptoms of depression during menopause include:

Persistent sadness or low mood: Feeling sad or down most of the day, nearly every day, for an extended period.

Loss of interest or pleasure: A noticeable decrease in interest or enjoyment in activities that were once pleasurable, including hobbies, social events, and sexual activity.

Changes in appetite or weight: Experiencing a significant increase or decrease in appetite, often accompanied by unintentional weight gain or loss.

Sleep disturbances: Insomnia (difficulty falling asleep, staying asleep, or waking up too early) or hypersomnia (excessive sleepiness or sleeping too much).

Fatigue or loss of energy: Feeling consistently tired, drained, or lacking energy, even after adequate rest.

Difficulty concentrating or making decisions: Struggling with focus, memory, or decision-making, which can affect work performance and daily activities.

Feelings of worthlessness or guilt: Persistent thoughts of self-blame, guilt, or feeling unworthy, which may be disproportionate to the situation.

Physical symptoms: Unexplained aches and pains, headaches, or digestive problems that do not improve with treatment.

Irritability or anger: Increased irritability, frustration, or anger, sometimes over minor issues.

Anxiety or restlessness: Persistent feelings of worry, agitation, or nervousness.

Thoughts of death or suicide: Recurrent thoughts of death, dying, or suicide, including making plans or attempts.

It's important to note that not all women experiencing depression during menopause will have the same symptoms or severity. If you or someone you know is experiencing any of these symptoms, it's crucial to consult with a healthcare professional for an accurate diagnosis and appropriate treatment plan. Early intervention can help manage depression and improve overall well-being during menopause.

KNOWING THE DIFFERENCE

Distinguishing between normal mood fluctuations during menopause and signs of clinical depression can be challenging, as menopause itself is a time of significant hormonal and emotional changes. However, there are some key differences that can help you differentiate between the two:

Duration: Normal mood fluctuations tend to be brief and temporary, whereas clinical depression typically lasts for at least two weeks or more. If you are experiencing persistent low mood, loss of interest in activities, and other depressive symptoms that don't seem to improve over time, it may be a sign of clinical depression.

Severity: While menopause can cause mood swings, irritability, and mild feelings of sadness or anxiety, the symptoms of clinical depression are often more severe and pervasive. If your symptoms are affecting your ability to function in daily life, maintain relationships, or perform at work, it may be indicative of clinical depression.

Range of symptoms: Clinical depression is not just about feeling sad or low; it encompasses a range of emotional, cognitive, and physical symptoms. These may include feelings of hopelessness, guilt, or worthlessness, difficulty concentrating, changes in appetite or sleep patterns, and even thoughts of self-harm or suicide. If you are experiencing multiple symptoms like these, it's more likely that you may be dealing with clinical depression.

Consistency: Menopausal mood fluctuations can often be linked to specific triggers or events, such as hot flashes or sleep disturbances, and may vary throughout the day or month. In contrast, clinical depression tends to cause a more constant low mood that is not necessarily tied to specific triggers or events.

If you suspect you may be experiencing clinical depression during menopause, it's essential to consult with a healthcare professional who can help assess your symptoms and recommend appropriate treatment options. Early intervention is crucial for managing depression and improving overall well-being during this transitional phase of life.

PREVALENCE

Research suggests that the risk of experiencing depressive symptoms increases during the menopausal transition. Some key facts include:

According to a study published in JAMA Psychiatry, the risk of depressive symptoms during the menopausal transition was nearly twice as high as the risk before menopause. The study examined over 1,300 women and found that the likelihood of experiencing a significant level of depressive symptoms was 1.97 times higher during the menopausal transition compared to the premenopausal period.

A study in the journal Menopause found that approximately 20% of women experience depressive symptoms during the menopausal transition. This percentage is higher than the estimated lifetime prevalence of depression in women, which is around 10-15%.

Research has shown that the risk of experiencing a first major depressive episode is higher during the menopausal transition than in the premenopausal period. A study published in the Archives of General Psychiatry found that the risk of developing a first major depressive episode during the menopausal transition was 4.5 times higher than before menopause.

Perimenopause, the period leading up to menopause, is particularly associated with an increased risk of depression. A study published in Psychological Medicine found that perimenopausal women were more than twice as likely to experience significant depressive symptoms compared to premenopausal women.

It's important to note that the prevalence of depression during menopause can be influenced by various factors, including genetics, lifestyle, overall health, and individual sensitivity to hormonal changes. By recognizing the increased risk of depression during menopause, women and healthcare professionals can take proactive steps to monitor and address depressive symptoms during this transitional period.

WAYS TO HELP

There are various ways to help women experiencing menopausal depression. It's important to consult with a healthcare professional to determine the most appropriate treatment plan based on individual needs. Some of the common methods to address menopausal depression include:

Hormone Replacement Therapy (HRT): HRT involves replacing the declining estrogen and progesterone levels during menopause to alleviate menopausal symptoms, including depression. It may be prescribed as estrogen-only therapy or a combination of estrogen and progesterone, depending on a woman's specific needs and medical history.

Antidepressants: Selective serotonin reuptake inhibitors (SSRIs) and serotonin-norepinephrine reuptake inhibitors (SNRIs) are commonly prescribed to treat depression during menopause. These medications can help balance neurotransmitters in the brain, improving mood and emotional well-being.

Psychotherapy: Cognitive-behavioral therapy (CBT), interpersonal therapy, and other forms of psychotherapy can help women cope with the emotional challenges and life changes associated with menopause. Therapy can provide valuable tools for managing stress, improving communication, and building resilience.

Lifestyle changes: Making healthy lifestyle choices can have a significant impact on mood and overall well-being during menopause. These changes may include regular exercise, a balanced diet, maintaining a healthy weight, getting adequate sleep, and practicing stress reduction techniques like meditation, yoga, or deep breathing exercises.

Social support: Developing a strong support network is essential for emotional well-being during menopause. Women can benefit from connecting with friends, family, or support groups, where they can share their experiences, learn from others, and find encouragement.

Alternative therapies: Some women may find relief from menopausal depression through alternative therapies such as acupuncture, massage, or herbal remedies like St. John's Wort and black cohosh. It's important to consult with a healthcare professional before trying any alternative therapies, as they may interact with medications or have potential side effects.

Nutritional supplements: Some studies suggest that certain supplements, such as omega-3 fatty acids, vitamin D, and B vitamins, may help improve mood and alleviate depressive symptoms during menopause. Consult with a healthcare professional to determine if supplements may be helpful and appropriate for your situation.

Consult with a healthcare professional: It's crucial to keep an open line of communication with your healthcare provider and discuss any changes in mood or emotional well-being. They can help monitor your symptoms, adjust treatments as needed, and provide referrals to mental health professionals if necessary.

Remember that each woman's experience with menopause and depression is unique, and what works for one person may not work for another. It's important to explore different treatment options, stay patient, and be proactive in seeking help to manage menopausal depression.

NATURAL SUPPLEMENTS

There are several natural supplements that have been suggested to help with depression during menopause. While some women may find relief from these supplements, it is important to consult with a healthcare professional before starting any new supplement regimen. Here are some natural supplements that have been studied for their potential effects on depression during menopause:

St. John's Wort: St. John's Wort is an herbal supplement that has been used for centuries to treat mild to moderate depression. It is thought to work by increasing the availability of neurotransmitters like serotonin, norepinephrine, and dopamine in the brain, which are involved in mood regulation. Some studies have shown St. John's Wort to be effective in alleviating depressive symptoms, but its effectiveness specifically for menopausal depression remains unclear.

Omega-3 fatty acids: Omega-3 fatty acids, found in fish oil and some plant-based sources, have been shown to support brain health and improve mood. They may help alleviate depressive symptoms by reducing inflammation and promoting healthy cell membrane function in the brain. Some studies suggest that omega-3 fatty acid supplementation can be beneficial for people with depression, including those experiencing menopausal depression.

Black cohosh: Black cohosh is an herbal supplement that has been traditionally used to treat menopausal symptoms, including hot flashes, night sweats, and mood swings. Some studies have shown that black cohosh may help improve mood and reduce anxiety during menopause, but more research is needed to confirm its effectiveness for menopausal depression.

Vitamin D: Low vitamin D levels have been associated with depression, and some studies suggest that vitamin D supplementation may help improve mood in people with depressive symptoms. As vitamin D deficiency is relatively common, particularly in older adults, supplementing with vitamin D may be beneficial for overall health and mood during menopause.

B vitamins: B vitamins, such as folic acid, vitamin B6, and vitamin B12, play essential roles in brain function and neurotransmitter synthesis. Some studies have suggested that supplementing with these vitamins may help improve mood and reduce depressive symptoms in certain individuals, including menopausal women.

Please note that while these natural supplements may provide relief for some individuals, their effectiveness varies, and not all supplements are suitable for everyone. It's essential to consult with a healthcare professional before starting any new supplement regimen, as they can interact with medications or have potential side effects.

COMMUNICATING WITH HEALTHCARE PROVIDER

Effectively communicating with your healthcare provider about depressive symptoms during menopause is crucial for receiving appropriate care and support. Here are some tips to help you discuss your concerns:

Be honest and open: Clearly express your feelings, symptoms, and concerns. Don't downplay or minimize what you're experiencing, even if you're unsure whether it's related to menopause or clinical depression.

Keep a symptom journal: Document your symptoms, including their frequency, severity, and duration. This information can help your healthcare provider understand your situation better and identify any patterns or potential triggers.

Note how symptoms impact your life: Describe how your depressive symptoms are affecting your daily functioning, relationships, and overall quality of life. This information can help your healthcare provider assess the severity of your symptoms and determine the most appropriate treatment options.

Share your medical history: Provide details about your personal and family medical history, including any previous episodes of depression, anxiety, or other mental health issues. Also, mention any other health conditions you may have and medications you're taking.

Discuss lifestyle factors: Talk about your sleep patterns, diet, exercise habits, and stress levels. These factors can impact your mental health and may be relevant to your treatment plan.

Ask questions: Don't hesitate to ask your healthcare provider any questions you may have about menopause, depression, or treatment options. Seeking clarification and understanding can help you make informed decisions about your care.

Express your preferences: Share your thoughts and preferences regarding treatment options, such as therapy, medication, or lifestyle changes. Your healthcare provider can then tailor a treatment plan that aligns with your preferences and needs.

Follow up: Stay in regular contact with your healthcare provider to monitor your progress and adjust your treatment plan as needed. Don't hesitate to reach out if your symptoms worsen or if you have concerns about your treatment.

By openly discussing your depressive symptoms and providing comprehensive information, you can help your healthcare provider better understand your situation and work together to develop an effective treatment plan.

SUPPORT

Supporting a loved one experiencing depression during menopause can be challenging but is essential to help them navigate this difficult period. Here are some ways you can provide support and resources available for family members and friends:

Be empathetic and understanding: Acknowledge their feelings and validate their emotions. Understand that menopause and depression can be challenging, and it's normal for them to feel overwhelmed, frustrated, or sad.

Educate yourself: Learn about menopause, depression, and their symptoms to better understand what your loved one is going through. This will help you provide appropriate support and guidance.

Offer a listening ear: Encourage your loved one to share their feelings and experiences and listen without judgment. Sometimes, simply having someone to talk to can be incredibly helpful.

Encourage professional help: Gently suggest seeking help from a healthcare provider or therapist who specializes in menopause and mental health. Offer to help them find a suitable professional or accompany them to appointments if needed.

Help with daily tasks: Offer assistance with day-to-day tasks that may become overwhelming, such as cooking, cleaning, or running errands.

Encourage healthy habits: Support your loved one in maintaining a balanced diet, engaging in regular exercise, and practicing good sleep hygiene. These habits can improve mood and overall well-being.

Be patient: Understand that recovery from depression may take time and that your loved one's progress may be slow or non-linear. Offer ongoing support and encouragement.

Resources for family members and friends:

Mental health organizations: Many national and local organizations provide information, resources, and support for individuals dealing with mental health issues and their families. Examples include the National Alliance on Mental Illness (NAMI) and Mental Health America.

Support groups: Look for local support groups for caregivers or family members of individuals experiencing depression or menopause-related issues. These groups can offer valuable information, resources, and peer support.

Online forums and communities: Numerous online platforms and communities focus on mental health, menopause, and caregiver support. These can be helpful sources of information and connection with others who share similar experiences.

Books and articles: Many books and articles provide valuable insights and guidance for supporting loved ones with depression or going through menopause. Educate yourself by reading these resources.

Workshops and seminars: Some organizations and healthcare providers offer workshops and seminars on mental health topics, including supporting loved ones experiencing depression or menopause-related issues.

By being patient, understanding, and proactive in offering support, you can help your loved one navigate the challenges of depression during menopause and work towards improved mental well-being.

DURATION

The duration of depressive symptoms during menopause can vary greatly from person to person. Some women may experience depressive symptoms for a few weeks or months, while others may experience them for several years. Some women may have no symptoms of depression at all.

It's also worth noting that menopause-related depression may occur at any point during the menopausal transition, including perimenopause (the period leading up to menopause) and post menopause (the period following menopause). However, some studies suggest that women are at a higher risk of experiencing depressive symptoms during perimenopause, with rates of depression increasing by 2-4 times.

COMMUNICATION

Deciding whether to discuss your menopause depression with your husband is a personal choice, and there is no right or wrong answer. However, it can be helpful to have a supportive partner who can understand what you're going through and offer emotional support.

Here are some tips on how to approach the conversation with your husband:

Choose the right time: Make sure to pick a time when your husband is available and not distracted by other tasks. Avoid having conversations when you're both tired or stressed.

Be honest and direct: Explain to your husband that you've been feeling down or depressed lately and that you suspect it may be related to menopause. Be honest about your symptoms and how they are affecting you.

Share information: Provide your husband with information about menopause and depression so that he can better understand what you're going through. You can also share information about the available treatments and how he can support you.

Listen to his response: Give your husband the opportunity to ask questions and express his thoughts and feelings. Listen actively and try to understand his perspective.

Seek professional help together: Consider seeking professional help together, such as counseling or therapy. This can be an opportunity for both of you to learn more about menopause and depression and to work together to find solutions.

RECOVERY

Depression during menopause is a medical condition that can be effectively treated with the right approach. With proper diagnosis and treatment, many women can overcome depression and go on to lead happy, fulfilling lives.

There are several treatment options for depression during menopause, including medication, psychotherapy, and lifestyle changes. Hormone replacement therapy may also be effective in some cases. Your healthcare provider can work with you to develop a treatment plan that is tailored to your specific needs and goals.

It's important to note that recovery from depression during menopause is not always straightforward, and it can take time to find the right treatment approach. However, with patience, persistence, and support from loved ones, many women are able to overcome depression and regain their sense of well-being.

It's essential to seek medical attention if you're experiencing symptoms of depression during menopause. Untreated depression can have significant negative impacts on physical and mental health, but with proper treatment, many women can effectively manage their symptoms and enjoy a better quality of life.

STIGMA

The stigmas surrounding menopause and depression can create significant barriers to seeking help, which can have serious consequences for women's mental health and well-being. Here are some examples of how these stigmas can cause harm:

Belief that menopause is a natural process that women should be able to handle without difficulty: This stigma can make women feel like they are supposed to be able to handle the challenges of menopause on their own. As a result, women may feel ashamed or embarrassed to seek help when they are struggling with depression or other symptoms of menopause. This can delay diagnosis and treatment and make it harder for women to manage their symptoms effectively.

Perception that depression is a weakness or a personal failing: This stigma can make women feel like they are to blame for their depression, or that they are somehow flawed or defective. This can lead to feelings of shame, guilt, and self-blame, which can make it harder for women to seek help and may prevent them from getting the support they need to manage their symptoms.

Misconception that depression during menopause is a "normal" part of aging: This stigma can make women feel like they should just accept their symptoms as a natural part of the aging process, rather than seeking help to manage their symptoms. This can delay diagnosis and treatment and can make it harder for women to manage their symptoms effectively.

Concerns about the side effects of medication: This stigma can make women reluctant to take antidepressants or other medications to manage their symptoms. This can prevent them from getting the help they need to manage their symptoms and can delay their recovery.

Fear of being perceived as "crazy" or emotionally unstable: This stigma can make women feel like they will be judged or stigmatized if they seek help for depression or other mental health issues. This can make it harder for women to seek help and may prevent them from getting the support they need to manage their symptoms effectively.

Overall, these stigmas can prevent women from seeking help and can delay diagnosis and treatment of depression during menopause. This can have serious consequences for women's mental health and well-being, and it's important to recognize these stigmas and work to overcome them. Seeking help and support for depression during menopause is essential for promoting recovery and improving quality of life.

There are several things that women can do to address the stigmas surrounding menopause and depression:

Educate themselves: One of the most important things that women can do is to educate themselves about menopause and depression. By learning about the symptoms, causes, and treatment options for depression during menopause, women can become better equipped to manage their symptoms and advocate for their own mental health needs.

Talk to their healthcare provider: It's important for women to talk to their healthcare provider about any symptoms they are experiencing, including depression. Healthcare providers can offer guidance on treatment options and can help women to identify resources and support that can be helpful.

Seek out support groups: There are many support groups available for women going through menopause or experiencing depression. These groups can offer a safe and supportive environment for women to share their experiences and receive emotional support from others who are going through similar challenges.

Challenge the stigmas: Women can also help to challenge the stigmas surrounding menopause and depression by speaking out and raising awareness. By sharing their own experiences and advocating for better education and resources, women can help to reduce the shame and stigma associated with these issues.

Practice self-care: Finally, women can take steps to practice self-care and prioritize their own mental health and well-being. This might include things like getting regular exercise, eating a healthy diet, practicing mindfulness or relaxation techniques, and engaging in activities that bring joy and fulfillment.

Overall, it's important for women to take a proactive approach to managing their mental health during menopause and to not let stigmas or misconceptions prevent them from seeking help or accessing the support and resources they need.

WORKPLACE/CAREER

Depression during menopause can have a range of effects on a woman's work life, including:

Decreased productivity: Depression can cause a lack of energy, motivation, and concentration, which can result in decreased productivity and work output. Women with depression may struggle to complete tasks on time, may make mistakes or oversights, and may find it difficult to focus on work-related activities.

Increased absenteeism: Women with depression during menopause may miss more workdays than usual due to their symptoms. This can be due to physical symptoms like fatigue or insomnia, as well as emotional symptoms like sadness, anxiety, or irritability. Frequent absences can lead to missed opportunities and decreased productivity over time.

Difficulty with decision-making: Depression can make it harder for women to make decisions or think clearly. This can impact their ability to perform job duties effectively, particularly in roles that require strategic planning or problem-solving. Women with depression may struggle to identify solutions to work-related challenges, may have difficulty prioritizing tasks, and may experience indecision or self-doubt.

Strained relationships with colleagues: Women with depression may find it harder to engage with coworkers or may struggle to maintain positive relationships with colleagues. This can be due to emotional symptoms like irritability, mood swings, or withdrawing from social situations. Strained relationships with colleagues can make it harder to collaborate effectively, may impact job satisfaction, and can contribute to a sense of isolation or disconnection at work.

Higher risk of job loss: In severe cases, depression during menopause can lead to job loss or forced retirement. Women with depression may struggle to keep up with work demands, may experience conflicts with colleagues or superiors, or may find it hard to maintain the level of performance expected of them. Job loss can have long-term financial and emotional consequences, including reduced income, loss of benefits, and a sense of purposelessness or loss of identity.

RELATIONSHIPS

Depression during menopause can have a complex and multifaceted impact on a woman's relationships. Here are some additional details on how depression can affect relationships during menopause:

Strained communication: Depression can make it harder for women to express their emotions and communicate effectively with their loved ones. Women with depression may feel withdrawn or irritable, which can make it harder to share their thoughts and feelings with their partners, children, or friends. This can lead to misunderstandings, miscommunications, and a sense of disconnection or isolation.

Reduced intimacy: Depression can also impact a woman's desire for intimacy or sexual activity. Women with depression may experience a loss of libido or difficulty feeling sexually aroused, which can strain romantic relationships. Partners may feel rejected or unloved, which can further exacerbate feelings of depression or anxiety.

Increased conflict: Depression can also contribute to conflict within relationships. Women with depression may experience irritability, mood swings, or outbursts of anger, which can cause tension and conflict with loved ones. Partners may feel like they're walking on eggshells or may struggle to understand their loved one's behavior, which can further strain relationships.

Social isolation: Depression can also lead to social isolation, as women may withdraw from social activities or events. This can make it harder to maintain friendships or engage in leisure activities with loved ones. Social isolation can exacerbate feelings of depression and loneliness, which can further impact relationships.

Caregiver burden: Women with depression during menopause may also experience a sense of caregiver burden, particularly if they have responsibilities for caring for children, elderly parents, or other loved ones. This can lead to feelings of guilt or overwhelm, which can further exacerbate feelings of depression and anxiety.

Overall, depression during menopause can have a significant impact on a woman's relationships. It's important for women to seek help and support for their symptoms in order to manage their depression effectively and minimize the impact on their relationships. This may include working with a mental health professional, engaging in self-care activities, and seeking support from loved ones.

JOURNALING

Journaling can be a helpful tool for managing depression during menopause. Here are some ways that journaling can help:

Emotional processing: Journaling allows women to process their emotions in a safe and private space. This can help women work through difficult feelings of sadness, anxiety, or anger that may be contributing to their depression.

Self-reflection: Journaling can also help women reflect on their thoughts and behaviors. Women may gain insights into patterns or triggers that contribute to their depression, which can help them develop coping strategies.

Gratitude: Practicing gratitude can help combat depression. Women can use journaling to write down things they are grateful for, which can help shift their focus to positive experiences and emotions.

Goal-setting: Setting goals can also be helpful for managing depression. Women can use journaling to identify goals for themselves, whether it's improving their mood, increasing physical activity, or working on their relationships. Writing down goals can help women stay accountable and track their progress over time.

Self-care: Finally, journaling can be a form of self-care. Taking time to reflect on one's emotions and experiences can be a calming and therapeutic activity, which can help improve overall well-being.

Helps manage stress: Menopause can be a stressful time, which can contribute to depression. Journaling can be a helpful way to manage stress, as it provides a way to process and release negative emotions. Writing about stressful events or emotions can help women feel more in control of their feelings and reduce the impact of stress on their mental health.

Provides a sense of control: Menopause can be a time of transition and change, which can feel overwhelming. Journaling can provide a sense of control and structure during this time. By setting goals and reflecting on their experiences, women can gain a sense of purpose and direction, which can help combat feelings of depression and hopelessness.

Helps identify patterns: Journaling can help women identify patterns or triggers that contribute to their depression. By reflecting on their emotions and experiences, women may notice recurring themes or situations that make them feel worse. This information can be helpful in developing coping strategies or making lifestyle changes to better manage their symptoms.

Encourages self-compassion: Journaling can be a form of self-compassion. By writing down their thoughts and emotions, women can validate their experiences and be kinder to themselves. This can help reduce feelings of shame or self-criticism, which can contribute to depression.

Enhances self-awareness: Finally, journaling can enhance self-awareness. By reflecting on their emotions and experiences, women can develop a deeper understanding of themselves and their needs. This can help women better advocate for themselves and make choices that support their mental health.

In summary, journaling can be a helpful tool for managing depression during menopause. It can provide a way to manage stress, gain a sense of control, identify patterns, practice self-compassion, and enhance self-awareness. Women may consider incorporating journaling into their daily routine to support their mental health during this time of transition.

ANGER

Anger is a common emotional symptom that women may experience during menopause. While not all women will experience anger during this time, those who do may find it disruptive to their daily life and relationships. Here are some details about anger during menopause:

Hormonal changes: Hormonal changes during menopause can contribute to mood swings, including anger. Fluctuations in estrogen and progesterone levels can affect the levels of neurotransmitters in the brain that regulate mood, leading to emotional instability.

Psychological factors: Menopause is also a time of transition and change, which can contribute to feelings of stress and anxiety. These emotions can build up over time and lead to anger.

Relationship issues: Menopause can put a strain on relationships, which can contribute to anger. Women may feel misunderstood or unsupported by their partners or family members, leading to feelings of frustration and anger.

Coping mechanisms: Women may also turn to unhealthy coping mechanisms, such as alcohol or substance use, to manage their emotions during menopause. These behaviors can exacerbate feelings of anger and lead to further problems.

PREVELANCE

It's difficult to provide an exact number on the amount of women who suffer from anger during menopause, as anger during menopause can manifest in different ways and may not be reported or diagnosed in all cases. However, some studies have estimated that up to 23% of women experience mood swings or irritability during menopause, which can include anger. It's important to note that anger is a normal emotion and can be experienced by anyone, regardless of age or gender. However, if anger during menopause is causing disruption to daily life or relationships, it may be worth discussing with a healthcare provider.

AFFECT ON LIFESTYLE

Anger during menopause can have a significant impact on a woman's lifestyle, as it can affect her relationships, work, and overall well-being. Here are some potential effects that anger during menopause can have on lifestyle:

Relationship problems: Anger can lead to conflicts and strain in relationships with partners, family members, and friends. It may also make it difficult for women to communicate effectively and resolve issues. Anger during menopause can have a significant impact on relationships, as it can lead to conflicts and strain in personal and professional relationships. Here are some additional details on how anger during menopause can affect relationships:

Communication problems: Anger can make it difficult for women to communicate effectively with others. They may be more likely to snap or say hurtful things, leading to misunderstandings and tension in relationships.

Resentment: If anger is not effectively addressed, it can lead to resentment in relationships. For example, if a woman feels unsupported or misunderstood by her partner, she may begin to harbor feelings of resentment that can build over time.

Distance: Anger during menopause can also lead to emotional distance in relationships. Women may withdraw from their partners or friends, feeling that they are not understood or that their anger is not validated.

Reduced intimacy: Anger can also affect physical intimacy in relationships. Women may be less interested in sex or feel too irritable or angry to engage in physical intimacy with their partners.

Misinterpretation: Others may also misinterpret a woman's anger during menopause. For example, a woman's partner may assume that her anger is related to something he has done, when it may be related to hormonal changes or other factors.

Work-related issues: Anger during menopause can also impact work relationships, as it can affect a woman's performance and relationships with coworkers. Here are some additional details on how anger during menopause can affect work relationships:

Decreased productivity: Anger can lead to decreased productivity at work, as women may have difficulty concentrating and completing tasks effectively.

Tension with coworkers: Anger can also lead to tension with coworkers, as women may be more likely to snap or become argumentative in response to stressors.

Misinterpretation: Coworkers may also misinterpret a woman's anger during menopause, assuming that it is related to something they have done or not understanding the underlying hormonal changes.

Work-related stress: Anger during menopause can contribute to overall work-related stress, which can further exacerbate the negative effects on work relationships.

Professional reputation: If anger is not effectively addressed, it can impact a woman's professional reputation and relationships with colleagues, potentially leading to missed opportunities or career setbacks.

To effectively manage anger during menopause in work relationships, women may benefit from seeking support from their employers or colleagues, practicing stress-reducing techniques, and seeking therapy or counseling when needed. They may also benefit from developing coping strategies to manage their anger at work, such as taking short breaks or practicing deep breathing techniques. By addressing anger during menopause in work relationships, women can maintain positive relationships with colleagues and achieve their professional goals.

Health problems: Anger can cause stress, which can have negative effects on a woman's physical health, including increased blood pressure, heart disease, and gastrointestinal problems. Here are some additional details on how anger during menopause can affect health:

Cardiovascular health: Anger can have negative effects on cardiovascular health, including increased blood pressure and heart rate. This can contribute to an increased risk of heart disease and stroke.

Mental health: Anger can also impact mental health, leading to feelings of stress, anxiety, and depression. These conditions can further exacerbate anger and contribute to overall poor health outcomes.

Sleep quality: Anger during menopause can also impact sleep quality, making it more difficult to fall asleep and stay asleep. This can lead to feelings of fatigue and reduced overall health.

Immune function: Anger can also have negative effects on immune function, making women more susceptible to illness and infection.

Chronic pain: Women experiencing anger during menopause may also be more likely to experience chronic pain, as anger can exacerbate pain and lead to a decreased tolerance for pain.

Increased stress: Anger can lead to increased stress, which can impact mental health in a variety of ways. Women experiencing anger during menopause may feel more anxious, overwhelmed, or irritable, which can make it difficult to manage daily responsibilities and lead to feelings of burnout.

Anxiety: Anger can also contribute to anxiety, leading women to feel nervous, restless, or on edge. This can exacerbate symptoms of menopause-related anxiety and make it more difficult to manage.

Depression: Anger can also contribute to depression, leading women to feel sad, hopeless, and unmotivated. This can make it difficult to enjoy activities, interact with loved ones, and maintain a positive outlook on life.

Emotional regulation: Anger can also impact emotional regulation, making it more difficult for women to manage their emotions effectively. This can lead to feelings of guilt or shame, as well as challenges in interpersonal relationships.

Overall quality of life: Anger can impact overall quality of life, leading women to feel less satisfied with their lives and more prone to negative thinking patterns.

DEALING WITH YOUR ANGER

Seek support:

Talking to a trusted friend, family member, or a therapist can provide emotional support and validation, which can help reduce feelings of anger and frustration. It can also be helpful to connect with others going through similar experiences, such as joining a menopause support group. Reach out to friends and family: It can be helpful to talk to people you trust about what you're going through. This might mean opening up to your partner, a close friend, or a family member. They may not have all the answers, but sometimes just having someone to listen and provide emotional support can make a big difference.

Join a support group: Consider joining a menopause or mental health support group. These groups can provide a safe and supportive space to share your experiences and connect with others who are going through similar challenges. Support groups can be found in person or online, and there are many resources available to help you find the right group for you.

Seek professional help: If your symptoms are interfering with your daily life, or if you're finding it difficult to manage your symptoms on your own, it may be time to seek professional help. This could mean seeing a therapist or counselor who specializes in menopause or mental health, or working with a healthcare provider to explore medication options.

Use online resources: There are many online resources available that can provide information and support for women experiencing menopause. These might include forums, chat rooms, or online support groups. It's important to remember to use caution when seeking support online and to make sure that any resources or advice you find are from reputable sources.

Remember, seeking support is a sign of strength, not weakness. By reaching out to others and finding ways to manage your symptoms, you can take control of your mental health and improve your overall well-being during menopause.

Practice self-care:

Self-care activities can help reduce stress levels and improve mood, which can alleviate feelings of anger. These activities can include getting enough sleep, eating a healthy diet, engaging in regular exercise, spending time outdoors, practicing relaxation techniques, and engaging in hobbies or activities that bring joy. Self-care is an essential aspect of managing menopause-related depression, anxiety, and anger. It involves taking intentional actions to promote your physical, emotional, and mental well-being. Here are some examples of self-care practices:

Exercise: Regular exercise can help to improve your mood and reduce symptoms of anxiety and depression. Choose an activity that you enjoy and aim to get at least 30 minutes of exercise each day.

Eating a healthy diet: Eating a balanced diet that is rich in fruits, vegetables, whole grains, and lean protein can help to support your physical and mental health.

Getting enough sleep: Aim to get 7-9 hours of sleep each night. Establish a regular sleep schedule and create a relaxing bedtime routine.

Practicing good hygiene: Taking care of your personal hygiene, such as showering, brushing your teeth, and washing your face, can help you to feel refreshed and renewed.

Engaging in hobbies and activities that you enjoy: Spending time doing things that you enjoy, such as reading, gardening, or painting, can help to reduce stress and improve your overall well-being.

Taking time for yourself: It is important to carve out time for yourself each day to relax and recharge. This can include taking a warm bath, practicing yoga, or simply spending time alone in a quiet space.

Self-care is an ongoing process and may require some trial and error to find what works best for you. It is important to prioritize self-care and make it a part of your daily routine.

Practice relaxation techniques:

Deep breathing, meditation, and yoga can help reduce stress and promote relaxation, which can alleviate feelings of anger. These techniques can be practiced daily or in response to feelings of anger or stress. Relaxation techniques can be a helpful tool in managing the symptoms of menopause-related depression and anxiety, including anger. Here are some common relaxation techniques:

Deep breathing: Take slow, deep breaths, inhaling through your nose and exhaling through your mouth. Focus on your breath and try to clear your mind of other thoughts.

Progressive muscle relaxation: Tense and then relax each muscle group in your body, starting with your toes and moving up to your head.

Yoga: Practicing yoga can help you to relax and improve your overall well-being. There are many different types of yoga, so it is important to find a style that works for you.

Meditation: Meditation involves focusing your attention on a single point, such as your breath or a specific word or phrase. This can help to calm your mind and reduce stress.

Guided imagery: Use your imagination to visualize a peaceful and calming scene, such as a beach or a forest. Focus on the details of the scene and allow yourself to become fully immersed in it.

Relaxation techniques can be practiced on your own or with the guidance of a mental health professional. It is important to find a relaxation technique that works for you and to practice it regularly in order to reap the benefits.

Seek professional help:

A mental health professional, such as a therapist or counselor, can help women develop coping strategies and work through any underlying emotional issues contributing to their anger. They can also provide tools for effective communication and conflict resolution. Seeking professional help is an important step in addressing underlying issues and managing difficult emotions during menopause. It is important to understand that seeking professional help is not a sign of weakness or failure, but rather a courageous step towards improving one's mental and emotional health.

A mental health professional, such as a therapist or counselor, can provide a safe and supportive environment to discuss difficult emotions and work towards developing healthy coping strategies. They can also offer insight and guidance on how to manage specific symptoms of menopause-related depression and anxiety.

It is important to find a mental health professional who is experienced in working with women going through menopause and who makes you feel comfortable and supported. There are a variety of options for seeking professional help, including private practice therapists, community mental health centers, and online counseling services.

Remember that seeking professional help is a proactive and positive step towards improving your mental and emotional health. It can help you to gain a deeper understanding of your emotions, learn effective coping strategies, and improve your overall well-being.

Address underlying issues:

Anger during menopause may be related to underlying emotional issues, such as unresolved grief or past trauma. Addressing these issues with a mental health professional can help reduce feelings of anger. Addressing underlying issues refers to identifying and addressing the root causes of anger and other difficult emotions during menopause. This involves taking a closer look at one's thoughts, feelings, and behaviors to determine what may be contributing to the anger.

Here are some ways to address underlying issues:

Identify triggers: Triggers are situations, people, or things that can cause an emotional response. By identifying what triggers your anger, you can take steps to avoid or minimize these triggers.

Challenge negative thoughts: Negative thoughts can fuel anger and other difficult emotions. Practice identifying and challenging negative thoughts by asking yourself if they are true, if they are helpful, and if there is evidence to support them.

Practice self-care: Self-care can help to reduce stress and improve mood. This can include getting enough sleep, eating a healthy diet, engaging in regular physical activity, and taking time for relaxation and leisure activities.

Seek professional help: If anger or other difficult emotions are significantly impacting daily life, it may be helpful to seek professional help. A therapist or counselor can provide guidance and support in addressing underlying issues and developing healthy coping strategies.

By addressing underlying issues, women going through menopause can better understand and manage their anger and other difficult emotions and improve their overall well-being.

Practice effective communication:

Learning to communicate effectively with loved ones and coworkers can help prevent anger from escalating into arguments or conflicts. Effective communication involves being able to express one's thoughts, feelings, and needs clearly and assertively, while also actively listening to and understanding the perspective of others. This can be particularly important for managing anger and other difficult emotions during menopause, as it helps to prevent misunderstandings, conflicts, and hurt feelings.

Here are some tips for effective communication:

Use "I" statements: When expressing your thoughts and feelings, use "I" statements instead of "you" statements. This can help to avoid blaming or accusing the other person, and instead focus on your own experience. For example, "I feel angry when you interrupt me" instead of "You always interrupt me."

Practice active listening: When someone else is speaking, listen actively and try to understand their perspective. This means paying attention to their words, body language, and tone of voice, and reflecting back on what you have heard to make sure you understand correctly.

Take a time-out: If you feel yourself becoming angry or overwhelmed, take a break to calm down before continuing the conversation. This can help to prevent escalating conflict and give both parties time to gather their thoughts and emotions.

Avoid using sarcasm or insults: These can be hurtful and escalate conflict and are not productive ways to communicate. Stick to expressing your own thoughts and feelings in a respectful way.

Use nonverbal communication: Nonverbal cues, such as facial expressions, tone of voice, and body language, can be just as important as the words we use. Be aware of your own nonverbal communication and try to interpret the nonverbal cues of others.

By practicing effective communication, women going through menopause can better manage their anger and other difficult emotions, maintain healthy relationships, and improve their overall well-being.

Practice mindfulness:

Mindfulness involves paying attention to the present moment without judgment. Practicing mindfulness can help women manage their emotions more effectively and reduce feelings of anger. Mindfulness techniques can be incorporated into daily activities, such as mindful breathing or body scans. Mindfulness is an ancient practice that has gained significant attention in recent years due to its potential benefits for mental and physical health. It is based on the Buddhist tradition of mindfulness meditation but has been adapted for secular contexts and can be practiced by anyone regardless of religious or spiritual beliefs.

Mindfulness involves paying attention to the present moment with a non-judgmental attitude. This means observing thoughts, feelings, and physical sensations as they arise, without getting caught up in them or trying to push them away. It also means accepting whatever arises in the present moment, without trying to change it or judge it as good or bad.

One way to practice mindfulness is through meditation, which involves focusing on the breath or a particular object of attention, and returning to that focus whenever the mind wanders. This helps to develop concentration and awareness of the present moment.

However, mindfulness can also be practiced in everyday activities, such as eating, walking, or even washing dishes. It involves paying attention to the sensations, thoughts, and feelings that arise during these activities, and staying present with them instead of getting caught up in distractions or worries.

Research has shown that practicing mindfulness can have a variety of benefits for mental and physical health, including reducing symptoms of anxiety and depression, improving cognitive function, reducing stress, and even boosting the immune system.

Overall, mindfulness is a valuable tool for managing anger and other difficult emotions during menopause, as it helps to cultivate greater awareness and emotional regulation, leading to a greater sense of well-being and fulfillment.

It's important to note that different strategies may work for different women, and it may take some trial and error to find what works best. Women should also talk to their healthcare provider to rule out any underlying medical conditions that may be contributing to their anger.

ANXIETY

Anxiety is another common symptom that women may experience during menopause. The hormonal changes that occur during menopause can affect the levels of neurotransmitters in the brain, which can contribute to feelings of anxiety. Additionally, menopause can be a time of significant life changes, such as children leaving home or retirement, which can also contribute to anxiety. Anxiety during menopause can manifest in a variety of ways, and the severity can range from mild to severe.

Symptoms of anxiety during menopause can include:

Excessive worry or fear about everyday activities or events: constantly worrying about the future, worrying about meeting deadlines or appointments, or fearing that something bad will happen.

Restlessness, irritability, and difficulty concentrating, feeling restless or on edge, easily getting frustrated or irritated, and having trouble focusing on tasks.

Physical symptoms such as muscle tension, trembling, sweating, and increased heart rate: experiencing muscle tension or headaches, trembling or shaking, sweating or feeling hot, and heart palpitations or racing heart.

Difficulty sleeping, including trouble falling asleep or staying asleep: difficulty falling asleep or staying asleep, waking up frequently during the night, or feeling tired even after a full night's sleep.

Panic attacks, which involve sudden and intense feelings of fear, with physical symptoms such as chest pain, shortness of breath, and dizziness: experiencing sudden and intense fear or terror, heart palpitations or racing heart, chest pain or discomfort, shortness of breath, dizziness or lightheadedness, and trembling or shaking.

Avoidance of certain situations or activities due to fear or anxiety: avoiding situations that trigger anxiety or fear, such as social gatherings or public speaking, or avoiding activities that used to be enjoyable.

Anxiety and Relationships

Anxiety can affect relationships in various ways, including:

Difficulty forming and maintaining relationships: Anxiety can lead to excessive worry, fear, and self-doubt, making it difficult to initiate and maintain relationships. This can result in feelings of loneliness and isolation.

Relationship conflict: Anxiety can cause individuals to overthink and overanalyze situations, leading to conflict in personal relationships. It can also cause individuals to become defensive, irritable, or easily agitated, which can negatively impact relationships.

Avoidance of social situations: Anxiety can lead to a fear of social situations, causing individuals to avoid them altogether. This can result in missed opportunities to meet new people and form new relationships.

Jealousy and insecurity: Anxiety can also cause individuals to feel jealous and insecure in their relationships, leading to mistrust and tension between partners.

Leading to communication problems: Anxiety can make it difficult to express thoughts and feelings clearly, leading to misunderstandings and miscommunications in relationships.

Triggering negative thought patterns: Anxiety can cause individuals to experience negative thought patterns and beliefs about themselves and their relationships, which can impact their behavior and interactions with others.

Affecting intimacy and sexual health: Anxiety can cause physical symptoms such as fatigue, muscle tension, and insomnia, which can impact sexual health and intimacy in relationships.

Contributing to codependency: Anxiety can lead to a dependence on others for emotional support and validation, which can result in codependent relationships and an unhealthy reliance on others for emotional wellbeing.

Anxiety and Career

The symptoms of anxiety, such as difficulty concentrating, lack of motivation, and fatigue, can affect job performance and productivity.

In addition, anxiety can also cause individuals to avoid certain tasks or situations, leading to missed opportunities for career advancement. It can also cause individuals to experience imposter syndrome, leading them to doubt their abilities and skills, even if they are qualified for the job.

Moreover, anxiety can also cause physical symptoms such as headaches, digestive problems, and insomnia, which can affect attendance and overall work performance.

Anxiety can also impact workplace relationships, causing tension and misunderstandings with colleagues or superiors. Women may feel isolated and unsupported, leading to further stress and anxiety.

Additionally, anxiety can affect a woman's career trajectory, as it may lead to missed opportunities, reluctance to take on new challenges, or even leave a job altogether. It can be difficult for women to balance their personal and professional lives while experiencing anxiety, which can further exacerbate the issue.

Anxiety and Physical Health

Anxiety can have both short-term and long-term effects on physical health. In the short-term, anxiety can lead to symptoms such as headaches, fatigue, muscle tension, and shortness of breath, increased heart rate, high blood pressure, muscle tension, and digestive problems. These physical symptoms can cause further stress and discomfort, exacerbating anxiety and making it more difficult to manage.

One possible explanation for the connection between anxiety and physical health is the activation of the body's stress response. When the body perceives a threat, such as a stressful event or situation, it releases stress hormones such as cortisol and adrenaline. These hormones can prepare the body for a fight or flight response, increasing heart rate, blood pressure, and respiration. Over time, chronic activation of the stress response can contribute to physical wear and tear on the body, increasing the risk for health problems.

Additionally, anxiety can interfere with healthy behaviors such as exercise, sleep, and nutrition. People with anxiety may have difficulty finding the motivation to exercise or may have disrupted sleep patterns. They may also turn to unhealthy coping mechanisms such as overeating or substance use.

Additionally, research has shown that anxiety can also weaken the immune system, making individuals more susceptible to illness and disease. Chronic anxiety can also increase the risk of developing chronic health conditions like cardiovascular disease, respiratory problems, and gastrointestinal disorders.

Things That May Help Your Anxiety

Exercise: Regular exercise is a great way to reduce anxiety symptoms. It can help to release endorphins, which are natural mood-boosters, and it can also help to reduce the physical symptoms of anxiety, such as rapid heart rate and shallow breathing. Aim for at least 30 minutes of moderate exercise, such as brisk walking, cycling, or swimming, most days of the week.

Relaxation techniques: Relaxation techniques, such as deep breathing, meditation, yoga, and progressive muscle relaxation, can help to calm your mind and reduce anxiety symptoms. These techniques can be practiced on your own or with the guidance of a professional.

Cognitive behavioral therapy (CBT): CBT is a type of talk therapy that helps you to identify negative thought patterns and replace them with more positive, helpful ones. It can be very effective for reducing anxiety symptoms, especially when used in combination with other strategies.

Hormone therapy: Hormone therapy (HT) can help to relieve menopausal symptoms, including anxiety. HT works by replacing the hormones that your body is no longer producing, which can help to stabilize your mood. However, it's important to discuss the risks and benefits of HT with your healthcare provider, as it may not be appropriate for everyone.

Medications: There are several types of medications that can be used to treat anxiety, including antidepressants, benzodiazepines, and beta-blockers. These medications can be effective, but they can also have side effects and should be used under the guidance of a healthcare provider.

Lifestyle changes: Making lifestyle changes can also help to reduce anxiety symptoms. These changes might include getting enough sleep, eating a healthy diet, reducing caffeine and alcohol intake, and avoiding stressful situations as much as possible.

It's important to remember that everyone's experience with anxiety during menopause is different, and what works for one person may not work for another. It may take some trial and error to find the strategies that work best for you, so be patient and persistent in your efforts to manage your anxiety.

Conclusion

Depression, anger, and anxiety are common experiences during menopause due to the hormonal changes that women go through. These symptoms can have a significant impact on a woman's quality of life, including their relationships, career, and overall mental and physical health. It is important for women to seek professional help if they are struggling with these symptoms, and to take care of themselves through self-care, relaxation techniques, mindfulness, and other coping strategies. With the right support and tools, women can effectively manage these symptoms and enjoy a fulfilling life during and after menopause.

References

North American Menopause Society. (2020). Menopause Guidebook. 9th Edition. The North American Menopause Society. https://www.menopause.org/for-women/menopauseflashes/menopause-resource-center

Santoro, N., Epperson, C. N., & Mathews, S. B. (2015). Menopausal Symptoms and Their Management. Endocrinology and Metabolism Clinics of North America, 44(3), 497-515. https://doi.org/10.1016/j.ecl.2015.05.001

National Institute on Aging. (2021). Menopause: Time for a Change. U.S. Department of Health and Human Services. https://www.nia.nih.gov/health/menopause

Harvard Medical School. (2019). Menopause: A Guide for Women and Those Who Love Them. Harvard Health Publishing. https://www.health.harvard.edu/womens-health/menopause-a-guide-for-women-and-those-who-love-them

Menopause and depression:
https://pubmed.ncbi.nlm.nih.gov/24951102/

www.ingramcontent.com/pod-product-compliance
Lightning Source LLC
Chambersburg PA
CBHW071036080526
44587CB00015B/2646